Praise for B

MW01283169

BORN TO MOVE

"I have a passion for running! This passion has led me to run and complete 34 ultra-marathons since 2010, averaging over five races a year. Since I returned to racing ultras in 2010, I have never had an injury that has prevented me from training or running my races. People may argue that feat is simply luck or the fact that I have been blessed with good biomechanics. Both of which could be true. But in all honesty, I attribute the majority of that success to Bryan Wisdom and the Fitness Together Mooresville team. Bryan's vast knowledge of kinesiology, biomechanics and corrective exercise, paired with their training philosophy is a perfect combination to achieve your fitness goals, injury free. This has been made evident to me time and time again as my body starts to break down from the abuse of running ultra-marathons. Bryan and team have always gotten me to the starting line, but more importantly, to the finish line as well.

"Thanks, Bryan! I appreciate your time and help!"

— Jeremy Alsop (Ultra Marathon Runner)

~~~~~

"When I saw a picture of myself in my mid 50's holding my grandson, I knew I needed to do something different. I was referred to Bryan from a friend who had great results with him and his staff.

"I've lost 35 pounds training with Bryan and his team. What's most impressive is working on my posture and movement. Bryan has helped my back pain and hamstring problems go away—I feel 20 years younger."

— Jim Johnston Business Owner

~~~~~

"I was recovering from a significant car accident, with a shoulder injury, when I first started working with Bryan. He helped me regain use of my arm and shoulder. I now have full range of motion and close to perfect strength.

"Thank you and your well-skilled team for helping me be successful and the best I can be."

— Alisa Nance M.D.

BORN
TO
MOVE

**The Ultimate Guide To Living A Pain Free
Active Lifestyle For The Rest Of Your Life**

BRYAN WISDOM

Born To Move

Copyright © 2017 by Bryan Wisdom, M.A. CPT

All rights reserved. No part of this book may be reproduced or transmitted in any form or by any means without written permission from the author. While they have made every effort to verify the information provided in this publication, neither the author nor the publisher assumes any responsibility for errors in, omissions from, or different interpretation of, the subject matter. The information herein is based on the opinions of the author and does not constitute a prescribed program. All persons should gain clearance from their doctor before beginning any type of exercise, nutrition, or supplementation program. The reader assumes all responsibility for use of information in the book.

Published in the United States of America

ISBN-13: 978-1542803113
ISBN-10: 154280311 X

Book interior design by Jean Boles
https://www.upwork.com/fl/jeanboles

DEDICATION

I dedicate this book to the dreamer. The believer in what is possible. To you that take courage in striving to become better. To my mentors that have guided me along my path. Those that choose personal development as a way to impact the world around them and make it a better place. Thank you to my family and friends that have supported me. Your support only helps me to further help others.

CONTENTS

FOREWORD

by Kyle Daniels

> *"His approach was a whole body approach to functional movement versus isolated site injury treatment."* —Kyle Daniels

"Getting second in the 2004 Catalina Classic paddleboard race was one of the best things that could happen in my life. That and a shoulder injury in 2005 taught me a big lesson. That lesson put me in Bryan's training room. With his experience and guidance, he designed a custom program that went beyond the physical, but also tapped into the mental strength I needed to get back into top race shape. (See Kyle's full story in Chapter 11 of this book.)

Bryan is ahead of his years in training knowledge and expertise. Even though we are on opposite coasts, I continue to seek his advice as I work through injuries and rebuild. A name like Wisdom is only fitting for someone who is on his way to being the premier functional fitness expert of our time."

INTRODUCTION

He was a sickly kid who suffered from asthma, intestinal problems and was quite frail. He wore glasses and struggled to live his first thirteen years on the planet. He was constantly sick. This boy was encouraged by his father, who knew the importance of a strong body. "Child, you are smart, but we need to strengthen your body. Your body will further extend your mind's visions and dreams."

He would take the encouragement of his father and transform his body and strengthen it to the point where he could keep up with any rough-riding cowboy, hunter, lumberjack or wrestler. That man would become the 26th president of the United States. Teddy Roosevelt says it about as well as anyone has. Get in the game. Take your shots and let things unfold. Your body is an important part of how well you impact the world, help your family, help the community and help and inspire others.

"It is not the critic who counts; not the man who points out how the strong man stumbles, or where the doer of deeds could have done them better. The credit belongs to the man who is actually in the arena, whose face is marred by dust and sweat and blood; who strives valiantly; who errs, who comes short again and again, because there is no effort without error and shortcoming; but who does actually strive to do the deeds; who knows great enthusiasms, the great devotions; who spends himself in a worthy cause; who at the best knows in the end the triumph of high achievement, and who at the worst, if he fails, at least fails while daring greatly, so that his place shall never be with those cold and timid souls who neither know victory nor defeat."

— Theodore Roosevelt

Thank you for opening this book. Enjoy. This has been a passion of mine for the last twenty-plus years. I'm a practitioner. I didn't want to come out and say this or do that before I had many years of experience to prove it. I've been in the trenches helping thousands of people over these many years. When you finish this book, if what I say resonates with you, then take action.

Get in the game. There's a game going on, and it's your life. Your choice how you play. Your time, dedicated to this endeavor or that. The great news is it's up to you. You have the power to transform your body and life. You can do it. Get clear, get focused, define your outcome, and begin now.

—Bryan Wisdom

If you would like more information my direct line is (704) 658-1522. Option two: Get a free copy of my Foundation Movements at FTLKN.com.

> *"If you can't take a huge step to begin with, take as big a step as you can, but take it now. Take it now."*
>
> **-Zig Ziglar**

.

CHAPTER 1

Walking Into the Greatest Golfer Of All Time

As I headed for the door, with the exercise training rooms behind me, I had one thing on my mind—fish tacos—and I ran right into him. Jack Nicklaus, the greatest golfer to ever play. As I looked up, I said "Hey, Jack" as one would to an old friend. He greeted me back kindly, "Nice to meet you. What's your name?" I said, "Bryan." I was surprised by his genuine kindness and interest in knowing who I was. Clients from all over North America would fly in to see us. Jack had been a client for years, but oddly, I hadn't met him yet because he would typically train with us during off hours. He was the only high profile client I hadn't met or worked with.

We had clients from Canada, Mexico, and even Europe and Asia come to see us. I was finishing my last day before leaving for the PLACE Corps. (Think Peace Corps.) Heading to work with kids in South Central Los Angeles for my three-year tour of duty.

To give you a window into the interesting world I was living in, where it was not uncommon to work with clients like Jack Nicklaus, Junior Seau, Trent Dilfer, John Lynch, Troy Brown, Luke Walton, and the one that was probably the most interesting of all, Tony Robbins. Tony Robbins might come into the clinic one day on a massive Harley, wearing leather biker chaps, or quietly walk into the training facility the next day, pondering and thinking to himself. It was so interesting to see so many people come from all over the place to receive exercise therapy from us. These were the typical clients that we were working with on a daily basis.

They would fly in from different parts of the country and ask us to treat them, work on their biomechanics, and give them passive and active functional and corrective exercises to work on their alignment and their bodies. We performed exercise therapy, analyzing posture and a number of functional tests and then come up with customized "menus" for each person to perform for one week. Then we would give them their next routine.

We also ran satellite exercise therapy training clinics in San Francisco, Dallas, Atlanta, Washington DC, New York, Connecticut, and a host of other locations. We would travel once a month to treat our national and international clients all over the United States and train our clients in Del Mar, California daily.

San Diego, California

The year was 2003, and this world I was working in was the Egoscue Method Exercise Therapy Company in Del Mar, California. I'd been working there for the previous five years. Pete Egoscue had created a great method for helping people to improve posture and movement. He had amassed a robust clinic with about twenty exercise therapists and a very interesting and devoted client base.

We would analyze client's posture and walking gait and then come up with a "menu" of corrective movements for the client to perform on their own for the next week. We were looking at the whole body and finding passive and active pose style exercises to get the body back to symmetry. We would analyze and help someone with severe lower back pain and work to improve their movement and balance, and they would feel better—often times almost immediately. It was truly an amazing learning/training ground for me.

Later that day we might work on a Pro Bowl NFL safety who uses his body as a human battling ram and needs the same help—passive and active exercises to regain body balance. Firsthand, I saw the results it made on people's bodies and on my own body and life.

During the summers we would run a pre-NFL training camp, and any athletes and functional clients that wanted to train in everything body balancing, designed by Pete, would come out for two weeks in July. Usually there would be twenty to thirty NFL players from different teams all over the league. I was one of the exercise therapists working for Pete, who personally trained me as an athlete and mentored me as one of his employees during those pivotal learning years in my career.

We would work with a stroke patient one minute, and the next we may be working with Tony Robbins. The great thing about the job was the range of clients that came in. Seven to ninety-plus years of age was the range I would work with, and the clients always had a story to tell. You might be asking yourself, "Why would so many clients from all over the country come to see us in San Diego, California? The answer to the question lies in my journey to find a movement expert.

A c t i o n Steps

What do you do daily/ weekly for exercise (specifically)?

What have you wanted to get back to or start doing?

_____

_____

_____

_____

_____

_____

_____

_____

_____

_____

_____

_____

_____

_____

_____

_____

_____

_____

CHAPTER 2

Bad News From a Doctor Changed My Life

> *"I broke at 32. I remained broken right through until I made the changes. I'm not broken anymore."*
>
> — Joe Cross: *Fat Sick and Nearly Dead*

I was sitting in the doctor's office, waiting to be seen by a local physician. The year was 1996. I'd finished my senior year of high school at Mira Costa High School in Manhattan Beach, California. Manhattan Beach was a hotbed for professional beach volleyball, and my high school was arguably the most decorated high school in the country, producing hundreds of Division 1 athletes, Olympic players, and a long laundry list of professional beach and indoor volleyball players.

My dream was to be a professional beach volleyball player. I believed in this vision even if the odds were stacked against me. My senior year, our high school team was 23-0 and won the national title for men's indoor volleyball. My plans were simple. Standing at 6'1", I would play outside hitter or setter, and after four years in college then head to the AVP—the Association of Volleyball Professionals. Players did it all the time at 6'2", and the coach of our high school team, who practiced with us daily, getting more reps for himself, was on the AVP with a handful of wins as a professional beach volleyball player. He would later win the 2000 Olympic gold medal in Sydney for beach volleyball.

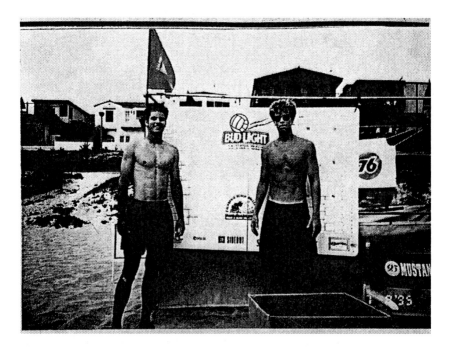

I had only one problem: my knees were trashed. I was broken. I knew this two years before, but I would ice and ibuprofen them sometimes three to five times a night, and I always found a way to train, work on my speed and jumping ability and lift weights. Finishing my senior year, the plan was to work on my volleyball game and have a great season at Orange Coast College in Orange County, California. The community college was one of the top men's volleyball schools, and I thought it was what I needed to polish my game before going to a Division 1 program. Everything was in place except for my knees.

Back to the doctor's office. When the doctor walked in, I explained this pain I had, which I had had for years. "I have tendonitis in both my knees that is manageable.

"What has gotten extremely worse, and seems to be debilitating, is my lower knee pain. Below my knees there is a bone pain that feels like someone is sticking an ice pick into my lower knees on both sides. This is a bit of a problem in a sport solely focused on jumping."

I waited for some wise words from the doctor. I figured there must be some kind of exercise training, some kind of therapy to fix these problems I faced, even surgery possibly. His response changed the course of my life. It was simple. He said, "The best way to get over this is... stop running; stop jumping."

What? Wait a second, I thought. A doctor in his fifties, he went to medical school, worked in his practice for twenty-plus years—that's the answer I get? I thought to myself, "Anyone could come up with a lame brain response like that. He didn't understand my plan." I was determined to become a pro beach volleyball player; jumping was part of the equation. Plus, no jumping for the rest of my life? I figured there's got to be a better way, a knowledgeable way. An exercise therapy program, rehabilitation, something out there for me. Where would I find it? That was the question. Not jumping or running for the rest of my life when I was only nineteen? That was just not good enough.

I quickly made an agreement with myself:

1. This guy doesn't even know HOW to help me.
2. The answer I was looking for was out there, but where? That was the question.

Big Dreams Shifted To Help Others

My dream to play professional volleyball evolved into, "I just want to be healthy." I was so committed to learning how to get healthy that I decided that if I could find a way to get myself better, I would use that knowledge to help others. At the end of the day, more important than playing professional sports was that I wanted to be able to move and play and be active for the rest of my life. This knee pain I had gotten was so severe I could hardly walk down stairs.

Bending my knees was beyond painful, jumping hurt, and landing was like a torture treatment. Every time I landed, I felt a sharp knife-like pain in both my knees. I could not go on like this as an athlete, and I could not enjoy a normal active life if I didn't find a solution to my knee problems.

Getting better consumed me. I have always loved to play sports, be active, to be outside. This was something I needed help with. I had felt the physical pain of my knees, and now the emotional pain of knowing that I could not do the thing I had wanted to do my whole life was a heavy blow.

What shifted in me was a strong empathy for others with body pain. I had always loved watching greatness. I could tell you everything you ever wanted to know about Michael Jordan. What took shape was the extreme desire to help myself and then help others. Heal the broken hearted, set the captives free.

I wanted to be the best I could be at making an impact in my 'soon to be clients' lives.' I love the quote from Zig Ziglar: "If you help enough people get what they want, you will get what you want." Helping others was a way for me to transcend my own struggles and focus on others. I felt liberated. I felt like the Grinch. My heart grew five sizes bigger when I made this shift.

My dream evolved to a dream bigger than myself. What type of training or healing arts would I go into? Physical therapy, chiropractic, acupressure, acupuncture, deep tissue therapy, or possibly become a physician? I was clear that whatever treatment could get me better after years of knee pain would be what I was going to commit to in order to help heal other people from their joint pain, limitations, and physical challenges.

Months after the meeting with my doctor I would end up spending a total of two-plus years doing different therapies and treatments. When the AVP orthopedic surgeon looked at me later and said, "I can do surgery on your knees," I asked him what was the percentage chance that this would help me.

"Fifty-fifty," he said.

I thought to myself, "Those are not good odds."

I later found myself two hours south of my home in Del Mar, California, sitting in front of Pete Egoscue. Pete, a former major in the Marine Corps, is a strong alpha-male personality. Growing up with my own father, who was a Vietnam veteran, I understood his personality and I pleaded with him for help by explaining the pain I had in my knees and the long list of treatments I had tried. I think he could sense my dedication to getting better and openness to his possible treatment. He began to explain, after taking posture photos of me, why my knees were bothering me. Skeptical, yet devoted to doing the passive posture exercises he gave me, I drove home with the "menu" I would do for the next two weeks before coming back to have him help me again.

What I didn't know at the time was the healing had started. Pete's idea of not looking at my knees solely, yet looking at balancing my whole body through kinetic chain alignment was a game changer. Getting better would take another three to six months of daily hard work, but for the first time, the cause of my knee pain made sense. After starting to feel relief after three months of doing the exercises, I felt empowered.

I made a major decision three months into my training with Pete and the Egoscue Method. One, I must learn this type of training and evaluating of clients. Two, I will work here when I finish my degree in kinesiology.

This type of *whole body balancing* is so different than the norm, so different than quick-fix training. It's more than just looking good. It's about a lifetime of health. My path had shifted. I wanted to help others move and feel better.

In my early years in the health and fitness business, I couldn't have been mentored by a better person than Pete. I would spend nearly five years learning and being mentored by Pete—first as a client and then becoming an exercise therapist for him from 1999-2003.

When I train clients, I am always looking on the long term rather than the quick fix. Lifetime joint and body health is not the hard-core-beat-the-hell-out-of-your body training. I want your body to last ninety years. For a body to function and last that long, body alignment and correct functional movement through space has to be a foundation. Everything builds up from here.

> *"Why do we fall, Bruce? So we can learn how to pick ourselves back up."*
>
> **— Batman Begins**

A c t i o n **Steps**

List any injuries past or current or any sore areas. How have they affected your workouts?

_____

_____

_____

_____

_____

_____

_____

_____

_____

_____

_____

_____

_____

_____

_____

_____

_____

_____

CHAPTER 3

The Hidden Secrets Many Fitness Professionals Don't Want You to Know

"There are no shortcuts—everything is reps, reps, reps. Everything I did, whether it is bodybuilding, making movies, or being governor, took a lot of work." **—Arnold Schwarzenegger**

Picture beautiful supermodel Brooke Burke-Charvet: brunette, long, lean, and vibrant. She is talking to the camera during a nice day somewhere in California. She is showcasing a slide board piece of fitness equipment and easily demonstrating how to use it.

Beautiful Super Model Makes It Look Easy

She slides side to side like an ice skater and then puts her hands down on the ground off the slide board and puts her feet on the slide board and facing down in a downward dog position, does a pike, kicking her butt in the air and then sliding both legs out and back, with her butt into the air.

She does it so gracefully one might think that this is an easy move. Furthermore, Brooke has had a few kids and has regained her near-perfect physique.

Anyone watching this infomercial might think that, "If she looks that great at forty-something, using that piece of equipment, then it will definitely help me. How much is it? Over a hundred dollars...no problem." You put your credit card in and voila. It comes in the mail seven weeks later because it was not immediately available.

What everyone that purchased this piece of fitness equipment didn't know is that Brooke was marketing this piece of equipment for the New Celebrity Apprentice with Arnold Schwarzenegger. Brooke had never used this product before. She may have used a slide board, but this was a prototype that she selected to market for the show out of five or six other fitness equipment pieces the day of the infomercial. She was marketing it for charity. The facts remain—this was not a piece of equipment she used every day for the last months or years.

Being marketed by a supermodel, it sold great. She's super fit. She trains all the time. She eats clean to my knowledge. It was a great ability to sell a product—but she doesn't even use it.

Why I've Been a Practitioner

For the last two decades I've been training clients. Many of my clients are in their 50-60's and often have some type of past or current injury and/or limited range of motion. It's collateral damage over time unless they have mindfully been doing healthy movement training. When one of my clients sits down with me for our strategy session, I point out the key areas we'll need to focus on to create change. Easy and quick is not part of the program.

I always like my clients to understand that it is possible to make a transformation. The hidden secrets that many fitness professionals and product sellers say out there is, "It's a quick fix; buy this ab roller, buy this DVD series, get this dancing DVD series, get this cowboy shuffle DVD series, get this quick-fix diet plan."

I think we know deep down that there is no quick fix. It doesn't exist. Truth be told, it will take a lifestyle shift over a prolonged amount of time.

Was It Really That Easy?

Matt Damon won the Academy Award at age twenty-seven for *Good Will Hunting*, and he looked like he was about twenty years old at the time. Many people thought, "Look at this kid... he's early twenties, and he's a natural. He's at the top of the acting community—so young, so quick." Just like the infomercials. This couldn't be any further from the truth. Damon had gotten into acting at thirteen years old and would work the next fourteen years of his life before we would see him on the podium at the Oscars.

Take Arnold Schwarzenegger, who created a fitness industry using weights to become a billion dollar industry. If you look at his best physiques, they were around years 1973-1975. He dominated the professional bodybuilding pro ranks. He got started at fourteen years old. It would take him seven years of laser focus to win Mr. Olympia and ten years to get his perfect physique. Ten years.

Now back to the infomercial industry, which is a billion dollar direct response industry. They do one thing great— they sell you products. The products can work if you use them, but make no mistake: Do them for three months and you'll see some results, but if you don't make it a lifestyle change, you'll be right back at square one. The other problem with many of these programs is that they are not customized for you. They don't take into account your health history or past or current injuries.

Furthermore, you may have potential injuries looming in the shadows that you don't see coming. Maybe you sit six to eight hours a day. Professional athlete or Jane Doe has a specific health history that needs to be known before training.

It is possible. It's possible for you to get into great shape. It's possible for you to move like you did years before.

Notice I didn't say you will; I just said it's possible. The catch is your transformation plan must be focused on your needs and adjusted to your further needs as you evolve. Every professional golfer knows this; that is why they have a swing coach even though they are professionals.

Let's be real here. You may have challenges, extra responsibilities, and that's understandable. Moving from where you are to where you want to be will take daily focus and daily tasks. Doable, but it's not about taking a pill, buying this DVD, buying this ab roller and you'll look like Jane Fonda, the fitness model, or Brooke Burke-Charvet, the fitness model.

You see, the real challenge that we all face that people often don't want to hear is that external daily responsibilities are putting extreme pressure and strain on our bodies. The very proper exercise and vertical loading demands are not being put on our bodies. This is not rocket science.

If someone said to a friend in the 1940s that they sit ten hours a day, five days a week, and then sit around on the weekends, it would be very clear that this behavior was not normal or healthy. They might say, "Are you sick? Are you dying? What's wrong?" Furthermore, sitting this long, it's crazy to think that one can offset this behavior with walking or light exercise two or three days a week. It's just a losing battle.

Did I Say Daily Movement?

You will need to do daily movement. It's a must. You will need to offset your sitting with vertical loading, cardio, strength training and body balancing exercises. It's not going to kill you. The good news is that it's doable, but you'll have to do it. It's not a quick fix. It's not a quick DVD series. It's not going to transform your body in thirty days. Let's think in terms of a year. You've got a year to transform yourself.

Also, the good news is that this book is written for someone who is in their forties to eighties and is open to doing something about the health of their body. If you have injuries, movement limitations, if you've not found success with the mainstream fitness classes, boot camps, cross-training, group workouts, personal training and gyms, read on. What you're going to read later is, "I believed it's possible to get better for myself even when I didn't know how I was going to do it."

> *"It's possible. It's possible. Just say that every day to yourself: it's possible. Because what does that do? See, it begins to change your belief system. So the way in which we operate, ladies and gentlemen, it's a manifestation of what we believe, what's possible for us."*
>
> **— Les Brown**

A c t i o n Steps

Change your belief system? *It's possible!* How are you progressing with your plans? It's not as easy as they say but it's possible. List workouts you want to get back to or start doing.

_____

_____

_____

_____

_____

_____

_____

_____

_____

_____

_____

_____

_____

_____

_____

_____

CHAPTER 4

Common Concerns and Injuries My Clients Face

> *"Pain is a sign we are in biomechanical compromise. That's the body's way of saying we are not moving correctly."*
>
> *"How many steps does it take to have a wear pattern if you walk like a duck?"*
>
> **—Kelly Starrett**

Back in college, I remember a roommate of mine saying, "I have back pain." My college roommate complained about debilitating lower back pain on this Friday night before a bunch of us were going out for dinner. I asked him, "What's going on? What's hurting?" He said to me, "I've been sitting for the last seven hours working on my computer, and I have shooting nerve pain going down my leg. I just can't go out. I know you guys want to, but I'm in too much pain."

If you could visualize his posture, his shoulders were rounded over, almost touching the keyboard. His head was about two inches from the screen, almost touching the computer. He had no lumbar curve; he had a reverse curve in his low back, and his lower back was being compressed, every disc one at a time.

Although he was in distress, I wasn't concerned because I knew a couple of posture exercises would snap him right back into a smile and he would be ready to go out to a restaurant. I had him do ten minutes of posture and positioning exercise to regain the curve in his lower back and get up and move around.

The funny thing to him was that his pain was gone.

The body is not designed to sit for ten hours a day. We are truly designed to move. If you're sitting in front of a computer screen for many hours a day, you may be in trouble.

Studies are showing links to many serious diseases as well as musculoskeletal problems related to sitting. We now have kids who won't jump, run and play outside. They are sitting for hours, playing video games online, offline, craning their necks to text friends and using social media on their cell phones—doing all of this for hours at a time. Kids are sitting during their crucial developmental years and adults are sitting and losing what function they once had.

Many of my clients have come into my studios with a long list of injuries and problems. They tend to have some kind of range of motion limitation at the very least. Whether it's a tight lower back from hours of sitting to decreased range of motion in both shoulders or an old sports injury that never fully recovered. More common past pain areas and injuries include low back pain, degenerative disc disease, back fusions, hip replacements, knee injuries, shoulder limitations, shoulder pain, shoulder replacements, neck pain, cervical fusions, and a host of others.

Common Injuries

It doesn't surprise me when a new client walks into my door and says they have been injured at a boot camp or cross training facility.

Throwing someone into high-impact personal training and group training day one is just crazy. No assessment of their movement and hoping they survive is a recipe for disaster. I'm not saying you won't see results in group training.

Again, there are people out there that really do care and are trying to make an impact on lives.

What I am saying is you want to learn how to move better in all aspects of your day-to-day life. Learning the correct body movements is more important than how many pull-ups or burpees you do. More importantly, are your joints getting healthier with your training? Are you strengthening your body for another forty to fifty years of movement?

One of my clients came in recently, and luckily his wife had prepped me on his spinal fusion and knee and neck injuries. However, when I asked him, "Do you have any injuries we need to know about?" his answer was "No, I'm fine."

The truth is, yes, you have some past movement limitations and compensations, and past injuries can be a future indicator of problems waiting for you. The only people I've ever come across that don't have any limitations are people that are aware of their body biomechanics and are performing functional movements on their bodies daily.

You want your trainer to ask a lot of questions about you. This is the time for you to be a little bit of a Hollywood star. Did you tear your meniscus thirty years ago in your high school football game? Or during your twenties during a Thanksgiving backyard game? Did you tweak an ankle wearing high heels walking down stairs? It's important and we want to know about you.

Standard group classes are designed for people with past knowledge of movement who do not have any current or past injuries and can correct themselves on their own during classes. No one is really looking out for you. It's really more of a survival of the fittest. "Do the exercise. If you can't, you're not trying hard enough," they'll say. Again, that's just crazy.

Training After 40?

What do you need to be doing after age forty? Some say cardio, others high-intensity beat-down workouts. Others will say nutrition. Some may say, "No, you're supposed to starve yourself in the morning and put butter in your coffee" or "No, it's lemon water. That's what you're supposed to do." I know this guy who lost thirty pounds drinking coffee and butter. People want the old Best Buy commercial: "I want it all, and I want it now." What works fast is usually not always best. You want a lifestyle change.

Let's say you're fifty. You want great health for the next thirty years of your life. What you don't want is great results for six months and then blow your back out doing a dead lift with maximum weight because you're trying to keep up with a twenty-seven-year-old muscle head in one of your cross training classes.

If you or your trainer are focusing on exercises like bench press and abs, and you're sitting eight to ten hours a day, you probably will only strengthen this detrimental rounded shoulder position. Surgeries for shoulder, knee, and hip are perceived to be easy oil change-type procedures. Doctors are changing our parts earlier and earlier.

Once we were changing out and replacing knees and hips when one was in their late sixties, maybe seventies. Easy for the surgeon but the rehab and range of motion and full function is critical.

Once the surgeon has done his work, you—the patient—have to retrain your body how to move correctly, and more importantly, create new patterns so you don't burn through the new joint you just got. The thing is, a replacement part does not have the longevity that a healthy human part has. There's a shelf life on your replacement part—years, maybe twenty. But let's be clear. If you go down that road, you want to take the best care possible of your body to optimize the joints you do have and decrease the wear and tear of the one you replaced. That only happens with better biomechanics, which equals better functional balanced movements through space.

As I'm finishing this book, one of my friends just had his hip replaced at age forty. That is a very young age to have a replacement joint. Our joints are designed to last a lifetime if we treat them with the right movement and mechanics and balance and load that they're designed to hold.

Shoulders are becoming a common replacement now that wasn't previously popular. The question that remains is, why we are cooking these joints so early? These joints are designed to last. What's going wrong?

With all these different pain points and concerns, how and why would you want to throw a client into a general high-intensity, high impact boot camp without evaluating past movements and limitations? I think that this is not a good idea. But people want results quick and are not thinking in the long term. How do the muscles look?

Arnold and His Buddies 25 Years Later

The famous movie, *Pumping Iron,* showcases Arnold lifting weights, getting ready for Mr. Olympia in 1975. I am a huge fan of what Arnold has meant to the fitness community and what he has accomplished in his amazing career. The movie is a docudrama of Arnold and his training buddies getting ready for the Super Bowl of competitions for the best bodybuilder in the world.

Arnold won. As he did many times. Watching the making of *Pumping Iron* twenty-five years later, the directors got many of the participants together. The sight of the guys was alarming. Many were so detrained they didn't look like they trained at all anymore. Keep in mind, these guys were the fittest looking bodybuilders on the planet. They were pioneers of the sport. What went wrong?

Muscles are only one piece of the equation. Injuries and challenges got in the way of their training. I could make a case that if the workouts are solely focused on muscle size and definition and not focused on functional movement of joints through space, one will run into problems.

Furthermore, putting max weight onto the muscles and joints when the joints are not working at optimal is a recipe for breakdown and injury. This is why when you see an older yoga teacher or Pilates teacher in their seventies and eighties looking great and moving so well, it makes sense they have been working on joint positioning and balance and muscle stabilization, not solely muscle hypertrophy (muscle growth).

What happens is a survival of the fittest process with hard-core, high-impact training. Some make it for a while, some quit, some injure themselves, and some never go back. The deck is stacked against you if you don't understand how to move better to help your body work at optimal levels. This knowledge is invaluable. What's probably even more important is that your fitness professional has the knowledge and applies proper movement training into their own workouts as well as their day-to-day clients' workouts.

If a client comes in to us during the intake process and says she has a lumbar back fusion, we have a game plan to balance her pelvis, work on low-and no-impact exercises and help her to understand how to move better on a daily basis. As fitness professionals, we need to know how she should be moving and transitioning, say, from up and down off the ground, and then we have to encourage her to make daily changes to move better in all movement patterns in daily life.

A c t i o n **Steps**

Change your belief system? *It's possible!* How are you progressing with your plans? It's not as easy as they say but it's possible. List workouts you want to get back to or start doing.

CHAPTER 5

At Age 45, 55, 65 Plus, How Do I Keep Up With People Half My Age?

"When we're young, we think we can live forever. We sometimes pay attention to our bodies and sometimes don't. We eat well and exercise, or maybe we don't. Either way, most of us survive, since the body has a curious habit of taking care of itself. But by the time we reach 40, we need to make a choice: is it time to give in or are we ready to beat the clock? Some people buy into the philosophy that you have a few good years before the next generation comes along and tells you to step aside.

(Sylvester Stallone continued on following page)

> *Don't believe that. The older we get, the smarter we get and the smarter we live. You can achieve extraordinary things into your fifties, seventies, and beyond if you really want to. It's that simple. All it takes is the desire to live better and the passion to feel more alive. It's that simple if you're prepared for it."*
>
> — **Sylvester Stallone,** *Sly Moves,* **page 3-4**

How do I keep up with women in their twenties and thirties doing group classes and boot camps when I'm in my forties, fifties, sixties-plus?" The question I often get is this, and the short answer is that oftentimes, you don't keep up. Some people can, but the truth of the matter is at forty-seven, fifty-seven, and definitely at sixty-seven, your ability to keep up with someone that's twenty-seven, that's never had an injury, is a bad bet.

How do you maintain a lifetime of health through fitness? This is a question you must answer for yourself. You must adapt, as they say in the Marine Corps. We all know an example of someone who had Navy SEAL type fitness or was a college athlete with a superior physique—and you see them now. They look like they spent the last years eating doughnuts for breakfast and fast food for lunch and dinner. What happened? The body is a tough cookie. It only listens to what you do, not what you say, not what you did years ago. The body doesn't care. What are you doing now and strategically planning for future workouts that matters?

Start Where You Currently Are

The first thing that we want to do is evaluate where you are now. Build on where you are now rather than have you try to keep up with somebody that's half your age, doesn't have an injury, and has experience in a certain class. We want to start with the baseline of where you are, what your past ability levels have been, what's your injury history or health history and then build up from where you are. Start at a certain point and build up. Think of your body as a base of a building, as its foundation. Put up the scaffolding, and floors.

This tends to be much more of a strategic approach compared to the general notion of "Let's throw thirty people into a class, make them all do the same workout." Well, scale the workout or not, meaning, we'll make it a little easier for this person and a little bit harder for that person. In the end, there's little to no evaluation of how somebody moves in a large group class.

Furthermore, there's no correction on making sure people do things right because, make no mistake, if you do certain exercises wrong, you may—and can—get injured. If you do a deadlift wrong, that's a great exercise to blow your back out.

"How do I keep up with people that are half my age in group classes?" one often asks. To recap, the answer is, you don't want to keep up. Even if you can, your goal is to get in the best shape you can be and not worry about how you used to be when you were twenty or thirty. Maybe you do get back to some of the success that you had in the past, but you want to train smarter. You want to be doing exercises that are strengthening your joints, that are putting your knees, your ankles, your hips, your shoulders in a better position. So you want to get a good workout and "pump," but more importantly, you also want to feel better after the workout.

If your joints are starting to hurt, if your knees are starting to hurt when you're doing a group class, you're probably doing something wrong. Furthermore, someone's probably not coaching you. They're not giving you the tools, the corrections, the guidance to make sure that you stay healthy. A client that comes in to me at fifty-seven, that's got some nerve pain in the back of his leg does not want to be keeping up with somebody that's twenty-five, that's never even heard of nerve pain, doesn't even know what it feels like to have nerve pain.

We want to get our clients in the best shape possible and the best position possible so they can be active and functional for the next thirty to forty years of their life.

If I Lift Weights Will I Look Like A Bodybuilder?

The second question is, does lifting weights make you look like a bodybuilder? I often get the question, "If I lift weights as a woman, will I look like a bodybuilder?" or "I don't want to lift weights because I don't want to look like a bodybuilder."

To start off, to look like a bodybuilder, a couple of things have to be in play. Lifting weights does not equal being a bodybuilder. A standard bodybuilder lifts oftentimes six days a week. They lift in terms of body parts.

Meaning, they focus on chest one day, back the next. They oftentimes will lift heavy weights, lower reps, and the rep count will be lower and the load (weights) are going to be heavier and heavier on the body. It's not uncommon to max and lift doing a very strategic and specific periodization program over an entire year to many years. It may take some bodybuilders ten years or more to get the professional bodybuilding physique seen in bodybuilding magazines.

The way that they eat is going to be massive calorie consumption oftentimes. If they're in any kind of competitive level of bodybuilding, most likely they're doing steroids, and PEDs—performance-enhancing drugs is definitely in play. When they get closer to their shows, they do cut calories and still maintain their lifting schedule. Steroid use is so common in professional and also amateur competitions that they now have a drug-free "Natural" competition bodybuilding series.

Unfortunately, I will get clients that say to me, "Well, I don't want to lift weights." That fallacy or myth will prevent them from any kind of success in transforming their physique because the normal common "Big Gym" mentality is "jump on a piece of cardio equipment and I'm going to look like this twenty-nine-year-old fitness model that's modeling for fitness magazines." It's just not true. Genetically speaking, there may be a few people out there that can look fantastic and do nothing at twenty-nine, thirty-nine, but that's especially equated with the type of foods that they eat. Nowadays, it's not very common.

The one thing that really transforms our physique is strength training, using weights and challenging the body, because what it does is force our muscles to have more of a training effect. As you lift weights, it breaks down your muscle, and builds it back up during proper nutrition, rest and recovery.

It creates much more of a lean, strong look, but it doesn't look bulky. Again, that is more of someone who is a seriously focused bodybuilder. Strength training not only builds lean muscle, it helps burn body fat, and if done correctly, causes the body to burn calories long after your workout is finished. When someone walks at a brisk pace and completes their walk for the day, their body stops burning calories. Makes sense. You finished your walk. The body rests. Strength training gets continued calorie burn long after your workout.

Lost Muscle As We Age

Strength training for people over fifty is increasingly important because of the muscle lost each year. We start losing muscle faster than we build it after about thirty. As we age to our fifties and sixties, our balance and motor control decreases. Lifting weights offsets this decline in muscle and reverses the tables.

Balance and Range of Motion

Strength training increases your locomotor balance, and if you are incorporating posture and body balancing exercises into your workouts, even further benefits will be seen with balance. Joint range of motion is equally important. As we lose muscle each year—due to our sedentary lifestyles, where sitting is a common daily position—our joint range of motion decreases. Our hips decrease in function and our shoulders decrease in overhead movements. This has a double-whammy effect. Not only are we getting weaker, we are also losing healthy joint movement.

While you probably won't be training high-impact, high-intensity training in your fifties and sixties and beyond, what's the alternative for you?

The importance is, number one, that we're keeping up with our training, and number two, that we also are setting a good example for ourselves. Trying to keep up with somebody who's half our age and doesn't have an injury, or trying to keep up with ourself, of how we used to be when we were in high school, does not make good sense.

What Did You Used To Do?

I oftentimes will get clients that will come to me and say, "Hey, I used to run 5Ks at X speed and time, and I used to do this and that." I say, "Well, when's the last time you ran a 5K?" That was something that this client had done consistently when she was seventeen; well, she's fifty-seven now. She hasn't run in over forty years. It's so important that we find ways to get back to being healthy, fit, and active, but that we're doing it in a manner that's making our body healthy and strong and physically fit and injury free. That is really an important piece to the puzzle.

I had a client who came in and said she wanted to lose about ninety pounds, and I said, "What do you do for activity?" She said, "Well, I used to play basketball and I was really good, and I played the three position and I loved it." That was thirty years ago. She hasn't picked up a basketball in maybe thirty years.

I love the fact that she's played basketball, so my first question was, "When's the last time you shot some hoops?" Probably a long time. Getting back to maybe just even shooting and doing some basic cardio, not going to play five-on-five, but just getting outside and going to shoot again might be something great for her to do.

The hard reality is that life gets busy for all of us and we forget what we love to do. We just stop doing it. You just have to remember and start DOING IT AGAIN. Your IT is whatever that IS for you.

What Makes You Come Alive?

She's doing cardiovascular training, and she's doing strength training, and she's making this a priority, but she's doing something that she used to love to do. Finding those things that used to make you come alive, that you loved to do, that you haven't done in a long time is important. Finding ways to get back to those things is even more important.

I'm as excited as ever when I do a Spartan race or a mud run because it reminds me of what it used to be like being a competitive athlete. Training and getting ready for different races that I do throughout the year—it's great. For me, I know it's not something that I'm going to win. I'm not going to win a Spartan race, and that's not being positive or negative. It's skill set. There are people who are much, much faster than I am, but I enjoy getting out there and challenging myself and running at times and climbing and jumping and hopping, and getting muddy and finishing the race.

My goal is always to challenge myself and finish the race pain-free, where my joints don't hurt. I'm doing a lot of training to work on my mechanics so that I'm able to exercise without pain. This enables me to move well, so that I can do a challenge like a mud run and still feel good. But I'm not trying to win the whole race. I'm trying to win my own race. I think it's just so important that as we get older, we're training, we're still doing some things that make us come alive, and we're also smarter about how we're training.

To conclude, you want to find exercises and activities that you love to do. You want to train smarter, you want to do high-intensity, lower-impact exercises as you get older, and still challenge yourself with some high-impact activities as long as your body feels good. Any kind of joint pain is pointing you in the wrong direction.

A c t i o n Steps

What are you doing daily to work on your Range of Motion of your body. How is that working? What areas need to get better?

_____

_____

_____

_____

_____

_____

_____

_____

_____

_____

_____

_____

_____

_____

_____

CHAPTER 6

High Impact Training, Extreme Workouts, It May Work...For Now?

"Due to most people's livelihoods—which is sitting—they literally forget how to move as humans. You see it all the time. You see people with canes, walkers, people in wheel chairs. It's like their brain shot off and they lose all those neural pathways. You see older people having trouble getting down on the floor and getting back up. One of the leading causes of death of people over seventy is falling. These are all things that happen because people literally just forget how to move because they don't move."

— Steve Maxwell, Fitness Pioneer

What's common right now is this proliferation of group training, which is good. Good people helping good people. There're a lot of health professionals out there that are trying to make an impact. What often is not happening, though, is a lack of evaluation of specific needs of each client walking into the door.

Why has group training exploded over the last five years? People like the community aspect of training. One fact I have learned with my clients is that shared suffering brings us together. We often do mud runs, weekly challenges, nutrition cleanses, hikes, and paddleboarding, to name a few.

I do think you can see results in many forms of training. Remember, I want you to move better. I want you to be coached and continue to practice better body awareness and proper range of motion of your body. If you find someone who is as passionate about your biomechanics as they are about exercise numbers, you have probably found a good fit.

The problem with high-impact, high-intensity group training, such as extreme cross training workouts and boot camps, is the survival of the fittest mentality. If the focus is more on beating someone else or trying to do your workout in as fast a time as possible, or do as many reps as you can, and form is not a priority, something's got to give.

Case in point, Joe who is forty-eight and played soccer in high school and had a minor knee injury and tight low back stiffness from his IT job is just looking to feel better day to day. He knows his back is becoming a problem due to the fact that his back is starting to bother him weekly, sometimes daily. He is losing the lumbar curve in his back due to his sitting schedule and inactivity. His lumbar spine literally stops moving as it used to in his fully functional soccer days.

He doesn't notice it other than the pain he feels in his back. He's heard about the latest high-impact group training in his town because his buddy has been going there for the last year and looks pretty good. Joe hasn't trained in about two years and he sees the ABC boot camp/cross-training company has a free two-week special. He figures, "I'll give it a try. What's the worst that can happen?"

Joe goes and realizes early on that his knee and lower back just don't feel right. It seems to get worse with each group training session. After the two-week trial, he surmises, "This isn't a good idea. I wish I could train like I used to, but I'm not a spring chicken anymore."

This could be a very different story if Joe was educated about correct movement and guided on how to improve his weak areas. As we get older, we must train smarter and be more focused on moving better. This notion is at odds with our sedentary/standard American lifestyle.

Or maybe you have Jane, who goes to an extreme cross training gym and loves doing a lot of the Olympic lifts. She jumped into a class and had someone show her some of the complex Olympic lifts and off she goes.

The unfortunate thing is that Jane has a nagging pain in her hip when she deadlifts. No real training was given on the movement, and during her workouts everyone is too busy to finish the level ten workout as quick as possible that no one is correcting Jane's poor lumbar posture that looks like a rounded road bike racer (think rounded turtle shell back position). She doesn't know it yet, but she is quickly wearing out/cooking her hip socket. She's on pace to have a hip replacement in a decade.

Moving Better and Feeling Better

We like to see our clients do some high intensity interval training but using lower impact training and improving movement in three planes of motion. Literally learning how to move better on a daily basis. This takes thinking about your movement as a daily practice. Something that is more important than your "workout." Because, make no mistake, you can work out and decrease your body's function over time if you are not teaching your body how to be a better mover. Your group membership is not going to be enough to make you a better mover. More focused training will be required.

The flip side to the above scenario is clients who do the same routine, like at Planet Fitness, where they're just jumping on a piece of equipment and walking on the treadmill for 30 minutes, texting their friends and looking at social media.

Interval Training Cardio Work

What we like to see our clients do is interval training or their cardio. They're not just doing the same intensity, but where they're training at certain levels while they're doing their cardio. You warm up for about 5 minutes then move your intensity to 60% of your max heartrate. Then you may go for 80% for a couple of minutes.

Let's say, for example, you're on the elliptical machine, where you're not pounding as much on your joints and you're going at an intensity level of 60% for a few minutes. Then you raise your intensity up to 80, even maybe 90% intensity for a minute, and then come back down to 60, then go back up to 80, go back down to 60, go back down to 80. Then cool down.

This is just a very, very basic high intensity interval training cardio workout, but one that is NOT going to be high impact on your joints, one that I like to recommend to our clients. We're still doing some high intensity interval training, but we're finding ways to do low impact, high intensity opposed to everything right now in the norm out there like high intensity, high impact, sprints, plyometrics, jumping, bounding, jump rope, pounding insane DVD's. I love a lot of that stuff, but it's not for everybody or for anyone every day, for that matter.

Now, again, you need to make sure that you're in good enough shape to do this. Clear this with a doctor, but you can do this on a bike, an elliptical. You can do this even walking, walking on a hill. You can do this on a treadmill, where you're not running, but using the treadmill as a hill. You're changing the intensity for periods throughout your entire workout, which raises your heart rate, then lowers your heart rate and tricks your body, breaking it out of that homeostasis.

What we discussed in this chapter was high-impact, high-intensity training, extreme workouts, boot camps, and cardiovascular training. People oftentimes are confused on where to start and ask, "Should I be doing this? Should I be doing this at this intensity?" Your workouts are best designed to be focused and sculpted around you and your needs.

When you're doing cardio, if you're doing a high-intensity boot camp, and you're being asked to do a bunch of burpees, and you tore your knee up or had a meniscus tear, and your knee is hurting every time you go down on a burpee, that is a bad bet. Listen to your body.

Long-Term Training/Long game

We've got to find ways to raise and lower your heart rate where it's focused more on low-impact training but still getting high intensity. That's the secret sauce and the secret component to having success over time because, make no mistake, you're going to hear this theme over and over in this book. We want you to be healthy and functional for the rest of your life. If you get in fantastic shape for a couple of years and you blow your neck out or rupture your disc in your back or blow out your knee, what's the use?

Shouldn't I Run?

The idea is long term. We're thinking about the next year of your life and the next thirty years—not a quick fix.

One-size-fits-all doesn't work. Another thing here is a lot of times people will ask me questions like, "I heard running is the best thing to get in shape" or "Running is the best thing to help me to lose weight." Running is great, but running may not be great for you. Running may be great for Jane, who just graduated from college and she ran in high school and she's got no joint pain and she feels fantastic. You may have had an injury that's been nagging—an ankle injury, Achilles tendonitis, a knee, a shoulder injury. That's not going to get you where you want to go. Try hiking at a quicker pace or trail running instead.

Running can be great if you feel great after you run. Are your joints and joint position good when you run. Are you running on different surfaces, hills, trails, asking your body to move in three planes of motion. You want your ankles to have full range of motion and be able to adjust to the different surfaces you provide.

There are multiple ways to raise your heart rate. Running in just one of many. We're going to look at ways we can raise your heart rate but focus on doing more low impact training, high-intensity training, and low joint impact. If you can do higher impact, that's great, but, again, you want to be smart about it. You want to be smart about the kind of impact training you're doing so that you're doing training for the rest of your life, not just a short term.

A c t i o n Steps

Focus on ways you can do cardiovascular training. What ways can you train and get your heart rate up without high impact training? List below.

_____

_____

_____

_____

_____

_____

_____

_____

_____

_____

_____

_____

_____

_____

_____

_____

_____

_____

CHAPTER 7

How Do I Become Pain-Free?

> *"Pain is a warning. Your body is saying stop. People forget how to move."*
>
> **— Steve Maxwell Fitness Pioneer**

What is the anatomical blueprint? What is functional 3-D movement through passive and active exercises? We have discussed many challenges people face on a day-to-day basis. When you open an anatomy book, certain symmetrical principles are very clear.

God designed our bodies for symmetry. When you look at the following picture—don't out think the room here.

BODY BALANCE BLUEPRINT

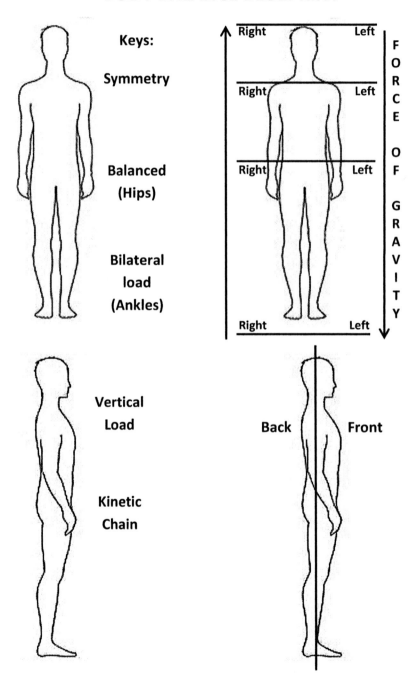

What do you notice? We have two hands, two feet, and two sides. What is critical is the body is balanced when you are looking at a front view of the body, where the chest stacks over the hips and the hips over the knees and the knees over the ankles.

From a side view, the ear stacks over the shoulders, hips over the knees, knees over the ankles, in a vertical load line. Most people do not stand static this way. Furthermore, most people don't go to this position naturally. So many external forces are literally physically, consciously and subconsciously, pulling us away from this position. When I'm evaluating clients initially, I want to know how well they vertically load.

Kids seem to understand this. When I watch my daughter move, she tires the most fit people. Running around after her for a day can be more tiring than doing a half marathon. Just try her movements. At two-and-a-half, she holds a full squat for fun for ten minutes at a time. She shifts from side to side. She crawls, jumps, hops, skips, run sprints around the kitchen—literally. Running on her fore-feet. All by lunchtime. The three planes of motion her body moves in is impressive.

Why We Lose ROM

We lose this range of motion and balance and load over time in our sedentary lifestyles. The standard American activity is sitting in front of a device. Sitting is the activity of choice. Craning our necks to read the latest Facebook post or text/read an email. Versus my daughter who is constantly moving, and for her to stay in one place for longer than about ten minutes is a major effort. If she is in one place, it's squatting and tinkering with Legos or one of her toy horses.

When I evaluate clients' movement, I am looking at how their bodies stack and track in static posture and then test/assess how well they move through space. How do their shoulders, hips, knees, and ankles move in a squat, lunge, in cross-body, cross-motor activities? When I watch my client do a squat, are they able to stay upright in their shoulders, keep lumbar extension in their low back? Are their knees tracking over their ankles and in line with their feet?

Oftentimes I see major hip strength differences from side to side. A client may have an elevated hip and be loading into one side as they lower into the squat. One side, even though they don't know it or how to fix it because it may seem too complicated, is taking over during the movement. Possibly the range of motion in one hip is so different than the other side.

So Joe from earlier decided to do squats with the Olympic bar and loads 135 pounds onto the bar. If his low back is so imbalanced and one side is taking over during the movement, compensation kicks in. Certain muscles work overtime.

NFL Wide Receiver Steve Smith

This is so clear when you look at someone who has had a major musculoskeletal surgery, like an Achilles tendon rupture. A specific example you could look at is with the wide receiver from the NFL, Steve Smith, who played for the Panthers—my local team—and the Ravens. Steve ripped his Achilles tendon off the bone. The compensation involved is severe, even with the best surgeon and best physical therapy. The body literally stops using one calf and leg for an extended period of time.

What's so clear about this example is if you look at someone who had an Achilles tendon rupture you can almost always tell. One calf will be noticeably larger than the other. I look at posture and movement every day, and believe me, anyone would notice the difference. Extreme compensatory muscles kick in, and the injured side gets weaker.

How Do You Compensate?

In a lunge we can spot major compensations. Some clients are unable to unilaterally (one side at a time) load their hip. They just don't have the range of motion in the hip socket because of extreme detraining and short, tight, dysfunctional muscles that support the hip, glutes, and hip flexors and stomach. Another example of compensation is lack of knee tracking during the lunge. The knee diving into the midline. Think knocked knees—the forward lunging knee is collapsing past neutral. This puts extreme load on the joint. You can spot these dysfunctions everywhere.

Why Should I Care?

We are not immune to these challenges. Someone asked me, "Why should I care about this?" Good question. The body is designed to last eight to ninety, even one-hundred-plus years. In the American culture we assume that we will live a long, healthy life. This is definitely a health bias that is simply not true. Some people are living longer, but many are not.

Serious musculoskeletal injuries are happening earlier and treatments to replace parts are happening as early as thirties and forties. Not to mention kids having heart disease. On the musculoskeletal front, our joints are designed to last us a lifetime if we take care of them. If we are so focused on doing a max deadlift, and say, lifting 300 or 400 pounds at twenty-five or thirty-five and we don't strengthen our anatomical body balanced position, our joints simply may not last.

Why should anyone care? My answer is you only have one body temple; if you care about making it last and function well, then function and body balance is essential.

Active 20 Years Later

I was getting ready to complete a half-marathon mud run called the Spartan Beast twenty years after I was sitting in the doctor's office as a college freshman. Thankfully, I didn't listen to his suggestion: "Stop running; stop jumping." Two of my rock star clients are by my side. I was nervous, probably for a lot of reasons. How would my knees hold up? The temperature was cold, and the race would cover some of the toughest terrain in South Carolina.

We would climb hills, crawl in the mud, swim across a creek, climb ropes, carry sandbags, jump over a fire, and run up and down some of the most even terrain around. We do these races like a bunch of navy seals: we stick together, help each other out along the entire course and always finish together.

As Kathy, Todd, and I crossed the finish line that day, I raised my arms in celebration. I got misty eyed and teared up for a second. The thought that I was helping my clients complete the race and the thought that I was able to run and jump and move all these years later was a testament to the notion that correct movement and biomechanics has had a huge impact on me and my clients' lives.

The problems many people face—injury, age, lack of training—are tough challenges indeed. The fact that I get to help others move better is truly a blessing that I am grateful for. Doing a mud run might seem like an extreme challenge or endeavor, and for someone else it might not seem extreme. But for me, the truth was I had trained for many years to get ready for that race. I had been doing mud runs for the last two and a half years before I did my Spartan Beast half marathon distance.

What Was the Cause of My Knee Problems?

Through much training, learning and body awareness, I found out the reason for my knee injuries had much to do with my lower leg biomechanics. I wore braces on my legs from one to two years old, and I have roughly a quarter inch leg length difference in my left leg. For many years I had no idea this leg length difference was throwing my entire body out of whack. I work daily on my body balancing exercises to improve my movement.

It always amazes me when one of my clients shares their past health victories. Deep down, they realize things have gotten out of hand and they don't know what to do to get themselves back on track. For me, it's always important to know the past movement patterns of my clients, what they've done and what they enjoy, what they love to do or used to love to do. Plus, it gives me an idea of any injuries that occurred over the years.

What are you passionate about?

What makes you come alive? Your likes and loves? I know it's not sitting in front of a computer for ten hours daily.

What makes you come alive? Write down three activities you used to do. Write down one or two activities you could do right now or this week to get back on track.

I want you to move better, transition better, be more balanced in your body. One of the things I look at is to analyze static posture—front, back view and sides posture. Then I analyze movement, walking, and gait. I also analyze kinetic chain of the body in different activities during a squat, a press, a pull, during a lunge, transitioning from up and down to the ground; these are critical movement pieces that are oftentimes overlooked.

Move It or Lose It

Nowadays, with the sitting culture that we live in, someone might sit ten to twelve hours a day. Maybe he or she goes for a walk two days a week or maybe he or she plays golf for the weekend once a week, or does a yoga class or a bar class or a boot camp.

The challenge with this is that the range of motion, mobility, and flexibility of the body deteriorates over time. Our bodies are truly a move-it-or-lose-it body.

As we move less, our range of motion decreases. As we move less, our muscles deteriorate and we get weaker. As we move less, our cardiovascular system does not have to work to its optimal levels. Quite clearly, movement is paramount. Daily movement is critical.

It Comes Easy For a Price

All these really are byproducts of becoming more of a functionally fit movement-centric human being. That is really counter-cultural, because nowadays, the common modus operandi is to do less. Find ways to get your food, meat, milk, vegetables, fruit, your bread, sugars, and your coffee.

All these things we don't have to work for. We don't have to do anything to get them. They're just there for us. We can quickly go through any fast food drive-thru and get anything processed, anything we like, with the snap of the fingers.

The unfortunate side of this is that as things come to us in an easier way, our bodies become weaker and weaker. The challenge is how we can offset this deterioration of our body.

Our heart becomes less efficient at pumping blood per beat throughout our bodies. This is why when you see someone who is really detrained, like someone who is 100 or 200 pounds overweight, when they walk up a small flight of stairs, their chest is bouncing back and forth at a rapid rate.

The heart is becoming weak and insufficient at pumping blood to the body, and because such a lack of blood is not pumping throughout the body, the heart increases the rapid amount of beats to keep up with the demand. In a nutshell, the heart just walked up a flight of stairs, but it's working like it just ran a 200-meter sprint at the Olympics at full speed.

We are really good at analyzing posture, movement, position, day-to-day range of motion, then coming up with a customized set of exercises and a program to help someone move better, become stronger, more balanced, decrease body fat, lose weight, and increase our heart health.

In conclusion, you want somebody who's able to look at your mechanics, look at your movements and help you to move better and help you to move without pain. Going through a workout where you have some soreness can be a good thing, especially if it's a muscle soreness and you feel like you're making progress. If you're continually feeling joint pain, that is a red flag that you really want to listen to.

Remember my story about my knees and finding my own success at getting over injuries? I was doing a mud run twenty-plus years later, which was a huge accomplishment because it asked me to do all the things that the doctor said I was not going to be able to do anymore: to run, to jump, to bound, to hop. All those movements are required in a mud run, and it causing my body to move through three planes of motion.

I've been training for years to keep my body balanced and able to perform at that level.

A c t i o n **Steps**

How can you become pain-free? What activities do you want to get back to? What areas of your body have affected your exercise? What posture deviations do you notice in your own posture?

_____

_____

_____

_____

_____

_____

_____

_____

_____

_____

_____

_____

CHAPTER 8

Confessions of a Fat Personal Trainer

> *"Food you eat is either making you healthier or sicker."*
>
> — **Dallas and Melissa Hartwig**, *It Starts with Food*

You know a little bit about my story and that I played volleyball in my formative years from eight to twenty years old. I jumped at the chance to play in a four-man beach volleyball tournament when I was about thirty-two. One of my good buddies who lived in Virginia Beach, our Nations East Coast center for Navy SEALs, asked me to come up and play in a beach volleyball tournament with him.

I gladly agreed. I was working a ton in my personal training business by training, managing my staff, and running the day-to-day operations of a small business. I was eager to play in this beach volleyball tournament and get some fresh air outside.

A Navy SEAL and Beach Volleyball

Me and my buddy and two of my other friends played in this four-man beach volleyball tournament. Chris, my Navy SEAL buddy, and Kip, another one of my buddies. Each team had a female; ours was Chris' fiancée, who became Chris' wife. Chris was a former Navy SEAL who had served our country, got injured in combat and had almost fully recovered from his injuries and was now back to work, working a very active job in the civilian world.

We played in the tournament, and my friend Kip made a funny comment, quoting Arnold Schwarzenegger. He said to one of his other friends on an opposing team of ours, "Before we started the tournament, I called my mother and I told her we had already won the tournament." I laughed. I didn't know how we would do but I felt pretty good about it, being that I was one of the ones who had played volleyball for many years.

As the four-man tournament went on, we won our different pool play games and then we won the tournament. I was feeling pretty good about myself. We took a picture of ourselves—myself, Chris, Kip, Carrie and the winning trophy. A picture tells a thousand words. Me, confident, the best player on the team. We won the tournament, and rightfully so; I had played volleyball practically my whole life. I was happy when we took the picture.

The Scary Truth about Pictures

What was so great about that picture was that I was standing right next to my buddy, Chris, who still looks like a Navy SEAL, and I realized something. *I'm running a fitness facility and I'm fat.* I had not trained consistently over the last two years. I had not been eating well. I had not been lifting weights consistently. I had not been doing cardio consistently and my body showed it.

What was great about that moment for me was that picture was a reality check. Secondly, before that picture, I might have told you if you asked, "How's your training and nutrition?" I might have said, "It's pretty good," but truth be told, it wasn't pretty good. I had started something I had never done through the years, started eating potato chips pretty consistently. I started drinking Dr. Pepper; I had not drunk soda since junior year in high school when I cut that out of my diet.

I had let in a number of little sabotaging nutrition adjustments over the last two to three years, and it finally caught up with me. When I won that tournament and took that picture, it was such a slap in the face. It said, "Dude, you're not in shape. What are you going to do about it?"

How's Your Nutrition?

Oftentimes, I'll have clients that come in that are in that same situation. They come in and they're trying to lose 20 pounds, 50 pounds, 100 pounds. I ask them, "How's your nutrition? How's your diet?" What do they say? "It's pretty good." That answer will get you nowhere. Even if your diet and nutrition is really good, we can break it down and probably make a couple of tweaks and improve your performance and results.

Tony Robbins says, "What are the first three letters in diet? Die." Very few people like going on a diet. I think there's truth to that. The response, just like what I said years ago— "It's pretty good. I eat pretty well. I don't eat out much"— shuts the brain down. No thinking is required for this response and no plans to change can come from it.

Although people are coming in for weight loss, it's very uncommon that our clients are fully aware of what their day-to-day nutrition choices and the effects of those choices are on their body. Remember what we said at the beginning of this book? This is about me being honest with you and you being honest with yourself. The question: "Why am I not losing weight? I've been doing everything right. I'm exercising. I'm eating better."

It can be complicated and it's dependent on each individual, but there's some specific behaviors that I have found that are very effective in losing weight, and more to the point, having a lifestyle and transformation change.

Tips for Success

A couple of things that are going to set you off for success: number one, track your calories for at least seven days. The reason I make this suggestion number one is that it is probably the most important one and the one that's hard for so many people to do. We have found, with remarkable certainty, that if you track your calories, you eat better and you lose weight. If you track your calories, you make better choices. If you track your calories, you do lose weight.

Why Should I Track Calories?

Why do so many people fight this? So many people don't want to track. "I just don't want to do it. It's too much of a waste of time. I just don't have the time. It's too much for me." I think they fight this for a number of reasons, but the idea of tracking your calories for the rest of your life, many people just won't do it. That's why I like to say seven days. You can do it for seven days. If you're serious, you'll do it. Track your calories for seven days.

It gives us a framework of what you're eating. It gives us an idea of where to start. It gives us an idea to see what your go-to meals are. Then we can find and build off some of the things that are working and make adjustments with some of the things that are not working.

Macronutrient Breakdown

Number two, once you track your calories on your app—My Fitness Pal is a good one, or something similar to that—you want to look at a couple of factors. One, how many calories are you consuming? Two, what is the macronutrient breakdown, and what frequency are you eating?

Dr. Barry Sears, author of *The Zone Diet*, suggests a 30-40-30 diet. Meaning, 30% of your diet comes from protein, 40% comes from carbs, and 30% comes from fats. (The term *macronutrient* describes the chemical substances that provide calories for energy, including carbohydrates, proteins and fats. *Micronutrients* include the many essential vitamins and minerals required in smaller amounts. Nearly all foods, with the exception of items such as candy that provide only calories with no nutrients, provide some amount of both macronutrients and micronutrients.)

Now, this is per Dr. Barry Sears, *The Zone Diet.* However, 30% protein can be difficult to achieve, and it's very difficult to achieve on the standard American diet. Most processed foods are heavily loaded with sugars, starchy carbs and unusable, empty calories.

If you're not being mindful about trying to get a 30% protein intake, you probably won't hit it. The standard American diet is much higher in processed carbohydrates and processed sugars. Liquid sugars—sodas—are a good example of calories that are coming from foods your body is not going to be able to use for benefit.

Changing that componentry to your diet alone is going to help you. Getting your calorie count correct is going to help. Then the time of day that you eat is also going to help. Keep in mind, I suggest whole foods, vegetables, leafy greens, fruits, nuts, organic meats to be your staple.

Are Sodas OK If They Are Diet Soda

Mission critical is to get off all soda. Period. All soda, extra sugar or no sugar, both have zero nutritional value for the body. Don't kid yourself with diet drinks. The term "diet drink" is marketing tactics to get you to think this is somehow good for you. Skinny latte. Same difference.

The zero-calorie sweeteners have many synthetic chemicals in the drinks, and the body thinks that it is sugar and has a hormone response to your diet drink even if you aren't taking in calories. So what's the alternative? Yep...you guessed it—water. Now, you can do some fun things with sparkling water and lemon or lime. Unsweetened teas are another great option if you need a little caffeine. Teas and black coffee are also options.

Processed Foods

The hardest challenge many of our clients have is getting off dairy, processed foods, sugars, sugar drinks at Starbucks, added sugars in their coffee, added milk in their coffee. These things are great for plumping you up. They're great for making you fat. My suggestion, which is a great option, is doing something like the Whole 30 cleanse, doing an actual challenge with yourself for a certain amount of days to break the sugar addiction.

Is Sugar a Drug?

It's oftentimes said—and I believe this—that sugar sets off receptors in your brain when you eat it. Tests have shown the brain lights up, like the same effect as when you're doing cocaine. Sugar absolutely can be treated like a drug and one that's very hard to get off of. Doing something like a cleanse, a twenty-one-day cleanse, or doing a Whole 30 cleanse will help. It really gives you the opportunity to make a shift and start eating better. Plus, you will see weight loss progress quicker if you are truly making a change in how you eat.

If you feel like you're addicted to sugar, you probably are. If you can do a cleanse, coupled with strength training, cardio and nutrition—I'm not saying be perfect—you will start to crave healthy whole foods. Once you finish the cleanse, take note of how you feel. Why go back to your old ways when you feel so much better? Stay on a clean, whole food eating lifestyle.

Shoot to eat well about ninety percent of the time. Then you can let yourself go off the grid for a cheat meal once a week. If you follow this system, you will probably feel sick when you eat unhealthy food options. You'll remember why you don't eat that way anymore.

How I Fell For The Junk Food Trap

The rub is when you're not exercising, and when you're eating processed foods, when you're eating foods that are high in sugar, your body literally craves those more. The idea of getting off sugar in your coffee is difficult when your body is literally craving it.

These dietary changes can happen without you noticing it. I remember that in my twenties I never drank coffee. Water was my thing. One of my buddies got me into it when we were working early morning, training clients.

A coffee once a week became three, and then before you know it, I was drinking coffee with heavy cream and raw sugar every day. That compounded over two years with my inactivity—I put on about twenty pounds of fat. It was a very slow process.

Can I Drink Coffee?

Now I drink coffee, but I take it black. Nothing but the coffee. I understand that no sugar in your coffee is a tough switch to make, but it's worth it. You get used to it. My dad used to drink black coffee in the military back in Vietnam and another trainer buddy also suggested it to me and I finally made the switch. In a perfect world I might not drink coffee at all, but I have found that I do enjoy a good cup of coffee.

Your body stops craving sugar once you get off of it for an extended period of time. Then you can use it as a treat: "I'm going to have a piece of cake at this birthday party, but it's going to be a certain size, and it's going to be on this day, and it's not going to be every day." You have a piece of cake once a month. That's fine. The goal really is that you're eating something like a 90/10 or 80/20, but really closer to 90/10 healthy choices. 90% of the time, you're eating healthy choices, 10% of the time or 20% of the time you're eating choices that are not healthy.

If you're getting back to a rhythm where you're consistently eating good foods the majority of the time, your body is going to crave more of a healthy good food option.

If you track your calories, if you make these adjustments, then you can really see. "Are things working or are they not working?" Some people say, "Things just aren't working. I'm not losing weight." Let's measure it. What are your key performance indicators—which they say in business? What are the key performance indicators for your health? What you eat specifically is a major factor on how your body functions.

A c t i o n Steps

Write down everything you ate yesterday.

Breakfast:

_____

_____

Snacks:

_____

_____

Lunch:

_____

_____

Dinner:

_____

_____

Drinks:

_____

_____

Put all items into a Nutrition App like MyfitnessPal.

Did you under eat or over eat for the day?_____cal. total.

What was your macronutrient breakdown?___/____/____.

CHAPTER 9

What Do I Look For in a Personal Trainer/Movement Expert?

"It is your birthright to live a pain-free and active life without limitations."

— Pete Egoscue

You want your trainer to have experience working with clients of many different age ranges. You also want to know if they're aware of terms like "corrective exercise," "scaling," and "adjusting workouts." A great question is, "Have you ever rehabbed a client of yours with a knee or shoulder injury like the one I have?" If the answer is no, that's not a good sign. Run for the hills to the next trainer.

Success Secret #1 Revealed

First, you want your training professional to ask a detailed set of questions about your health history, past injuries, and your past and current movement and exercise.

The truth is, yes, you have some past movement limitations and compensations, and past injuries can be a future indictor of problems waiting for you. You want your trainer to ask a lot of questions about you. It's important, and we want to know about you.

How we should train Scott, who is fifty-three and has a past shoulder injury, is different than how we train Zach, who is twenty-seven and has no shoulder problems and wants to increase his bench press. Often the challenge for guys at the gym is the fallacy of trying to keep up with the Joneses.

Scott goes in to train at his local community gym and has been off training for the last five years, or worse, twenty years, and he used to lift weights back in college. But at fifty-three, he decides it's time to get back to the strength training he once did. He used to play a little football and was pretty strong. He sees Bob Big Arms lifting 225 pounds bench-press—no problem. He thinks to himself, "I used to do that. I can keep up with that guy."

Big mistake. Scott lowers the weight, notices a strong pain in his shoulder, and gets off two reps. He goes in the restroom deflated. Not only was he not able to lift the weight he used to, he now has soreness lingering in his shoulder and struggles to lift his arm. He heads home and doesn't go back to the gym. "I learned my lesson," he says. "I need cardio. Someone on TV said that if I buy this elliptical-type machine, I can lose body fat and increase my muscle."

Success Secret #2 Revealed

Another great question to ask your potential fitness professional is, "What kind of nutrition program do you suggest to your clients?" "Nothing" is about the lamest answer any trainer can give. The trainer has a large portion of his or her clients that want to lose weight, increase muscle, and nutrition is a huge piece of the puzzle.

It would be like going to the gas station and needing gas for your car. You walk up to the counter because you have cash, and say to the clerk, "I'd like $50 on Pump seven." And she says, "We don't carry gas, but I'd be happy to sell you some chips."

Success Secret #3 Revealed

Another key point is you want your trainer to measure your body fat, your girth measurements, a strength test, cardio test, and weigh you and track your progress over the year. Ideally, they're assessing you every eight weeks at a minimum. They're going to notice your progress or lack of progress and be able to make adjustments along the way.

This is so important, because as a client is assessed, we know the real starting point.

Often when I ask a client how much they weigh if they have not been weighing themselves lately, that number on the scale is higher than what they think. They didn't notice the ten pounds they put on over the last months. Gauging your exact measurements and numbers lets us know where you are and where we want to go from here. What's more, when you see progress, we know how much progress you've made and also we know where we are headed.

Success Secret #4 Revealed

Does your trainer do a posture and movement assessment of you to gauge your strengths and weaknesses? You want someone to look at the symmetry of your body and see what is in alignment and what is not. If you sit eight hours a day at an IT job, the exercises we do will need to be specific to help you extend your body and activate and strengthen the muscles that shut off from being in that rounded, flexion position all day.

You want your trainer to watch your gait and score how your body moves through 3-D motion in a number of different exercises. Movement is a critical component to everything we do.

For example, one of the key exercises everyone knows about is the squat. Well, there is a correct way to do a squat to maximize the power posture of the spine, load the legs correctly, and track the knees and feet in the same plan. You want your trainer to look at a key movement like the squat and help you improve on it. This is just like having the old golf coach there to make suggestions on your swing plan.

Furthermore, the squat is one of the most important movements we make. It's one that you will need to make for the rest of your life. Think of getting on and off the toilet—it requires body control and lowering oneself to the seat.

Success Secret #5 Onboarding System

Does your trainer have an onboarding system that takes you from where you are to where you want to be? Are they assessing your body composition, putting you with a nutrition plan, giving you corrective exercises to work on your weak points, and giving you cardio prescriptions?

Look for a trainer that is putting all the pieces of the puzzle together for you and is encouraging you to take ownership of your health. You want your trainer to empower you to take your training seriously because it will take a focused effort to see the results you want. The onboarding system gives you the tools for success.

Success Secret #6 Revealed

Additionally, does your trainer have a background in fitness? Did they go to college for exercise science or kinesiology? Does your trainer have the education and certifications that are important when they are creating effective workouts for you? I like to see trainers with a four-year degree in exercise science or kinesiology and a personal training certification from a reputable personal training certification and be CPR/AED certified.

Two-day Certifications

Did you know there are a number of personal training certifications that can be accomplished in a weekend? You can become CrossFit Level 1 certified in two days and open up a facility if you wanted. That may be okay if you're leading a group of people with no prior injuries or performing safe and elementary exercises, but why chance it? Ask your trainer about his or her education and certifications.

Success Secret #7 Revealed: Walk the Walk

Finally, does your trainer walk the walk and talk the talk? Is your trainer setting a good example by being in shape? Running a business is not easy, even if it's fitness, but your trainer, whether they are an owner or employee, must be taking care of themselves. You may struggle with making fitness a priority, and that is the very reason you signed up or are interested in signing up.

When you look to your trainer, if they complain about being "TOO" busy to train, this will not consciously and subconsciously empower you to make the adjustments and sacrifices necessary to change. Your trainer's passion for running, lifting, fitness contests, races, or whatever they are into will inspire you. Make no mistake, you want a fit trainer that loves to help others.

I love surfing, mud runs, hiking in the mountains near my house, and a host of other activities. I have activities going the entire year. You want your trainer modeling healthy fitness behavior.

Red Flag Habits

There are red flag habits you want to steer clear of when hiring a trainer. Trainer Joe has real trouble with scheduling his clients. He doesn't use a scheduling software and needs to schedule his clients in different times each week. He has real trouble coming to work on time. Joe/Jane always has a 'great excuse.' My car wouldn't start, my cat had diarrhea (someone has really used that one on me), my alarm didn't go off, and on and ad nauseam.

Phone Use By the Younger Generation

Joe/Jane is constantly on his or her phone. They are looking at their phone as much as they are you. You get the sneaking suspicion they don't really give a crap about you. It seems that your trainer is not interested in your workout, and his or her attention to their phone is a clear example of that. Remember, it's not what someone says but what they do. You want them engaged and participating in your success in the workout.

Another distraction is Joe and Jane are often caught checking out the "hot chick/hot dude" in the gym. Again, you are not top priority. The funny thing is you are paying a lot of money for this girl/guy to pretend they care about your goals.

Your trainer keeps moving locations every couple of months. You start with him at one big box gym, and he moves to another big box gym, and then moves to his garage. Not ideal for you.

This Isn't My Real Job

This is a great one: Trainer Joe says, "This isn't my real job... I'm just doing it for the summer." Okay, but I'm paying you seventy-five bucks an hour to have you pretend to train me, and you have no problem taking my money.

Joe is a bartender at nights and trains some during the week. This is clearly just a temporary job for him while he finishes school. Quite frankly, I don't want to know if this isn't your thing. I want you committed to helping me—the client. Because the reality is, it's not the fact that Joe is still in school while he trains you; it's that he doesn't think this is his thing. Like he is going to greener pastures. It would be more inspiring if I knew Joe was giving this 100 percent while he is going through this phase of life. In a perfect, world you find someone who has made health and fitness a lifetime pursuit.

The Kiss of Death

The kiss of death would have to be the negative Nancy/Nick who finds a way to complain about something every time you train together. You think to yourself, "Maybe it's me." Don't be so hard on yourself; Nick/Nancy complains constantly, and you need encouragement, not bull crap complaints about their cat that had diarrhea the night before.

You want a trainer that cares about you every time they see you. They generally want to help you succeed. Ideally, your trainer has a heart for service and serving others. A trainer is allowed to have a bad day but not often.

It really is a job of motivation and encouragement. The funny thing about it is that even if I am having a bad day, my wife is nagging me, the kids kept me up all night, I always feel better when I focus on my clients when I come in and focus on how I can help them.

I quickly forget about my own temporary problems and focus on serving. This is really one of the coolest things about being a trainer. You will know if your trainer cares or not, and if you feel they are not invested in you, it's time to try someone or something else.

So, in conclusion, there are a number of factors going into finding a good personal trainer/movement expert, and understanding your movement, your mechanics, your body fat, looking at what you're eating on a day-to-day basis, looking at your cardio prescription, looking at what kind of strength training you've done in the past and what kind of strength training that we want to do in the future are all important components at getting you where you want to go.

Look for a trainer who embraces all the pieces of the puzzle of a wellness program: trainers who are performing body fat and body composition assessments, that are doing foundational, functional movements, that are helping you with the basic nutritional components, that are prescribing you cardio prescriptions and strength training on a consistent basis.

A c t i o n **Steps**

List two to three of the most important things you are looking for in a fitness professional? What kind of support and environment are you looking for?

_____

_____

_____

_____

_____

_____

_____

_____

_____

_____

_____

_____

_____

_____

_____

_____

CHAPTER 10

Younger This Year

"Remember your dreams. We're nowhere without them. When I was very young, I started to visualize what I wanted to be and even what I wanted to look like. Those visions started to come into focus in my 20s. Even facing financial obscurity, I had an insane dream. The one thing that never cost any money was being able to visualize where I wanted to go in my life. And here's the amazing thing: seeing myself as a success tricked my mind into believing I really was a success. That sort of thinking triggers winning streaks."

—Sylvester Stallone, *Sly Moves*, page 201

"People always came up to (me) and say, 'Why are you smiling? You're working out five hours a day. You're doing the same as the other guys, but the other guys have a sour face, they're pissed off that they have to do another rep or another set of something.' I looked forward to... I looked forward to another thousand reps of sit-ups. I looked forward to another 500 pounds of a leg press or squat. I looked forward to doing more and more curls until my arms fall off. Why? Because I knew that every rep that I did, and every set that I did, and more weights that I lifted, I get one step closer to turning that vision into reality. I was turned on by that. I was excited. I couldn't wait to get to the gym."

— **Arnold Schwarzenegger**

It Starts In The Mind

Arnold may seem extreme in his quote, but he created a scenario for himself that when he trained he got closer to his goals. Working out became fun and exciting. He focused on the benefits, not the strain and struggle.

So often a client will come to see me for the first time and say, "I hate to exercise. I just don't enjoy it." Some people enjoy it; others have attached such a feeling of pain and discomfort and suffering that they literally "hate" to do it.

The results are in and everyone knows it. Americans are officially obese. The recipe is simple. Eat processed food void of nutrients, eat foods high in sugar, and don't exercise and don't strength train and…. Americans are obese. Not one state in our country is fit when you run the numbers.

Why I bring this up is because we have to make a mind shift for any of this proper nutrition and physical activity to work. Eating healthy whole foods, eliminating processed foods from your diet (which you have to work at to do), and incorporating daily exercise and strength training multiple times a week will create change. For you to stick to any of these suggestions in this book, you will be required to shift your mindset.

An Injured Shoulder and the Race of His Life

It starts in the mind. I remember one of my clients and close friends I worked with back in Redondo Beach, California was getting ready for the biggest competition of his year and possibly the crowning moment of his career, The Catalina Classic. This is a thirty-two mile open ocean prone paddleboarding race (think face down on your stomach).

Kyle would be competing for his 5th title, but he injured his shoulder and did not compete the year before. He called me and asked if I would help train him in corrective movement and see if we could get him back in functional movement shape to race. I felt confident I could help him.

We began our work almost a year before his race, and I thought he could get back in movement shape, but getting back into paddle shape was going to be tough.

Furthermore, because of his shoulder injury, he was not able to put in as many miles as he usually would. His goal to win was clear from the start. We stayed focused and I noticed something as the year went along. He was moving without pain; we were able to load his shoulder and work on total body balance, regaining symmetry he had lost. Being the competitor he is, I could tell he might be ready to win this race again.

The Greatest—Jamie Mitchell

What gets better is that we found out about two months before the race that the best open ocean paddleboard racer of all time from Australia, Jamie Mitchell, would be competing in the race. For those of you who have not heard of him, this guy had not lost a distance paddleboard race in five years.

He was complimented by the greatest professional surfer of all time, Kelly Slater, saying, "What he has done is second to none." Kelly was referring to the ten years of dominance during which Jamie won the Hawaiian Molokai to Oahu thirty-mile paddleboard race every year for ten years straight.

Furthermore, Jamie was in his prime. This guy didn't lose races of distance over ten miles, and Kyle would need to regain balance and strength in his shoulder, need to train for the race, and then compete against the greatest competitor in outdoor watersports history.

To Kyle's credit he decided in his mind he would win. We were reading books that got his mind right, which further solidified this belief that he would win. I was encouraging this all the way, and I was amazed at the level of belief that he really felt like this was his race to win. He just decided. I knew I could help his body biomechanics, but this mind shift was amazing. As the race got closer, we would work on his movements and he looked and felt great. Shoulder was as good as new.

The race starts at 6:00 a.m. on Catalina Island, a very small island thirty-two miles from mainland Southern California. The open water is rough and cold, and conditions can be brutal in the Pacific Ocean. You have a rescue boat ride next to you to supply food and water throughout the race. The race is so long, each contestant must have boat help in case of needed rescue.

Kyle felt great as the race started; he and Jamie pulled away from the pack of racers after a couple of miles into the competition. Jamie and Kyle were alone for the next roughly 30 miles. They would exchange the lead back and forth, neck and neck. This became a battle of wills. Kyle would take a drink of water or take in a power bar and Jamie would pass him powering along. Jamie would take a quick food break and Kyle would power past him.

Mindset Meets a Lifetime of Hard Work

Kyle said he felt nearly exhausted with the pace of the race. Two miles out from the finish Kyle and Jamie were still neck and neck. Kyle felt like if this was his moment, now was the time to go for it. All the training, the focus, the mindset would be needed to pass Jamie and paddle the last two miles and not be caught by the best paddler in the world.

The James Allen quote we had practiced was running through his head: "Think strongly, attempt fearlessly, accomplish masterfully,"—and Kyle added, "Persevere relentlessly." He took off and pulled away from the machine. He kept going and going. He pulled away ten seconds, twenty, thirty seconds. As the last mile continued, Kyle pulled away further.

He would win and beat the unbeatable on an injured shoulder the season before. I was truly proud of Kyle for getting back to race shape, doing the work that was necessary to get back in the game. I'm most proud of how he believed he could do it even if it had not been done before. His mind was set. He believed and then went all in to accomplish his goal.

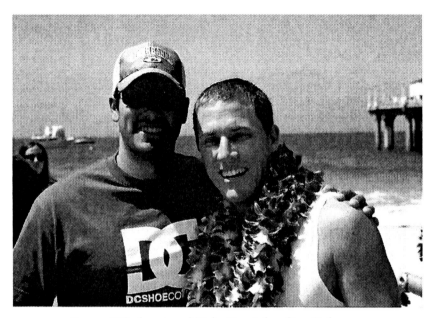

**Bryan Wisdom and Kyle Daniels after Kyle won
The Catalina Classic, Manhattan Beach, California**

Younger This Year

'Younger this year' starts in your mind. You must believe it's possible. The headline "To Lose Weight Fast" is popular. "Inches Melt Away," "Keep Burning," "Lose Weight in 21 Days," "90 Days to the New You." They're great headlines, and the great thing about them is they get people to take action and buy the DVD or infomercial or sign up for the membership.

The problem I have with them is it's a false narrative. Anyone who has trained for years knows, number one, it's going to take a lot of hard work. Secondly, it's going to take dedication and commitment over an extended period of time for you to see results for the long term.

One Year Is Needed

My goal for you is to accept the fact that it will take an extended amount of laser focus and extended commitment over time. So think a year.

No quick fix, no quick transformation, no quick diet. Better yet, think the rest of your life. Remember, diet—D-I-E. Because here's the thing, quick weight loss can equal quick weight gain. The body's a tough cookie.

One of my college professors explained it so clearly. Scientifically based, if it takes you six months to get into great shape, you can lose it twice as fast as you make progress. Twice as fast means in the real world if it takes you six months to get into great shape—shape that you love—in half the time you can lose almost all you accomplished. Just three months off. How often does that happen from maybe October, November, and December— off for family and the holidays, which is understandable.

And you lose all the weight loss and/or strength improve-ments that you gained. It just seems unfair, but it is fair. The truth over the myth is that you will need to take good care of your body for the rest of your life. Think lifestyle transformation long term. Throw out the quick fix mentality.

Do cleanses and jump starts work? They only work if you use them as a launching pad and go from a jump start into a continued lifestyle change and are committed to yourself. I have a client who is doing that exact same thing.

She's doing a nutrition cleanse and then is excited to dovetail that into a very consistent training program with strength training, nutrition, cardiovascular training, and corrective exercise.

The reason I titled this chapter "Younger This Year" is that I want you to wrap your head around the idea of focusing on your healthy lifestyle change for the next year, and I guarantee you will see transformation.

Turn Back the Clock

In conclusion, you're really turning back the clock. You're turning back the clock on your body. How you become younger this year is focusing this next year on getting in better shape, and that includes doing things that are going to make you feel better and move better, not just hard workouts. You're going to do exercises that focus on working on your posture, that are working on a healthy cardiovascular training program that's typically lower impact, working on strength training exercises that are less jarring on your joints but are still putting a load on your body.

A c t i o n Steps

How can you become pain-free? What activities do you want to get back to? What areas of your body have affected your exercise? What posture deviations do you notice in your own posture?

_____

_____

_____

_____

_____

_____

_____

_____

_____

_____

_____

_____

CHAPTER 11

How Do I Get Started?
Self-evaluation and Action Steps

> *"If you talk about it, it's a dream; if you envision it, it's possible, but if you schedule it, it's real.*
>
> — Anthony Robbins

California Surfing

Living nearly thirty years of my life in Southern California, I've always had a love for the ocean and water. I didn't know until I moved away from the ocean how much I missed it. I tend to be drawn to water sports. I love to surf and do multiple forms of surfing. The love for water caused me to move and live on Lake Norman.

I love the moment when you're surfing in a little bit bigger waves, and a big wave comes and knocks you down, deep underwater. As you go under and the pressure rises, it's a normal reaction to panic. It's a normal reaction for someone that's not used to being in the ocean to maybe swallow some water. I love these moments because I take a deep metaphorical breath and stay really calm.

As I'm going down, deep underwater, the white bubbles are gone and the water is darker, and I love this moment because it requires a sense of clarity, it requires a sense of focus often lost in daily life. The only option when I'm going deep underwater is to relax, take it on the head, and be clear of mind.

Calm and Clear of Mind

One task is before me: get to the surface. As I'm swimming back up and emerging, my mind is clear and there's only one thing I want to do—breathe. As I break the surface after being under the water for twenty or thirty seconds, there's an absolute sense of clarity when I come up. I'm back to reality. This is a clearing, an awesome moment. It's almost spiritual. It's the gift of life, and I'm back to reality.

Coming out of the water reminds me of that clarity of mind. Think of the time when you came out of the water, if you were swimming or you had to hold your breath underwater for an extended period of time. As you broke the surface how all you wanted to do was breathe. How you can be laser focused at getting your health where you want it to be. Make it a "breathe" type priority.

Be Really Clear

Think the same for your fitness. You're trying to get back into shape, and you're going to do it by being super focused on doing tasks to get you back in shape. Center that focus on doing daily movement and activity for a lifetime of health. Decide. Schedule it. "I will do daily movement and activity like I'll brush my teeth." Schedule your workouts and daily movement into your phone's calendar. Get it done.

Let's Get Started: Self Evaluation

How you get started. Self-evaluation action steps moving forward. First off, we want to talk about doing a self-evaluation so that you can see where you're starting from. For our clients, when we're starting out, we look at some key factors that are really important. Health history, we discuss their fitness activities, we cover their goals, and then we do four posture photos. We do a walking evaluation, we look at the kinetic chain of their body and their alignment, we do body fat measurements, we do strength tests, cardio tests, and we weigh our clients.

For you, I want you to think about doing a couple basic assessments to see where you start. I want you to get out your cell phone, go into your bathroom, put on a bathing suit, and what you're going to do is you're going to put your cell phone on record. Put your camera in a position where you can see your full view.

You're going to look straight ahead at the camera so you can see your full body. Front view facing straight ahead, side view, other side, and then back view. You're going to hold each position for ten seconds. Then you're going to analyze those posture views that we're going to talk about in a few minutes. *Turn to the Self-Assessment Chart and fill out your numbers for the rest of the assessment.*

Remember, we are looking at the anatomical blueprint and comparing our postural position to it. Are your shoulders level? Is one side higher than the other? Are your hips even? Are you knees pointing straight ahead? Is one pointing straight ahead and one pointing out or in? Are both your knees pointing in? Are your knees valgus (knocked-kneed) or Varus (bow-legged). Which direction are your feet pointing? Straight? In? Out? Make notes on the following page on what you see. Make notes on each measurement. You will measure these numbers every two months for the year.

SELF-ASSESSMENT CHART
Note Posture Findings in Each Box

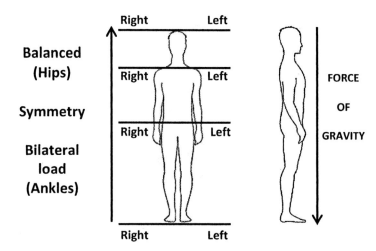

Tape Measure	2 Months	4 Months	6 Months	8 Months	10 Months	12 Months	Beyond
Waist							
Hips							
Weight							

Fundimental Tests	2 Months	4 Months	6 Months	8 Months	10 Months	12 Months	Beyond
Stork Stand							
Bird Dog							
Arm Glides							
Wall Sit							
Chair Squats							

The second thing you're going to do is to get your tape measure and measure your waist. Then I also want you to measure your hips. You're going to measure your weight, so stand on the scale and write your scale number down. Then, we're going to do a few functional tests.

Feel where your weight is in your feet. Is it toward your right foot or left foot? Now I want you to find a doorway or something very stable for balance, if needed, and you're going to lift your right leg like a stork. As you do the stork stand try to perform the exercise without assistance. If you need to hold the wall or door, do so. Your goal is to be able to stand on one leg without assistance. I want you to stand on one foot for twenty seconds.

Then switch sides and stand on the other leg for twenty seconds. Notice if you felt more balanced on one side or the other. Then we're going to go into a position called the Bird Dog on the ground. You're going to reach with opposites and hold for twenty seconds and notice if you felt any weakness lifting one side versus the other.

Now I want you to look at those posture photos. Do you notice that your shoulders are level? Are your hips level? Are your feet pointing straight ahead? Is one foot turning out more than the other? Is one knee turning out more than the other? Look at your posture. Now you're going to look at your side posture photos. Are your shoulders rounded? Is your head forward? Are your hips swayed forward? Then look at your back view. Do you see that your knees are knocking together? Are your feet pretty even? Is one foot turned out more than the other? Are your feet pronated? (think arches collapsed) Are your feet supinated? (think arches roll to the outside)

Once you look at these posture photos and once you've looked at your waist, your weight, and your hips and your stork stand and birddog, we're going to get started on transforming your body. We're going to measure these numbers and measure your balance and your movement over the next year. Every two months, we're going to measure your progress, and I want to see these numbers go down.

Daily Movement Guide Defined

Each day of the week you will have a workout to complete.

Daily: I recommend doing posture and body-balancing exercises called your *Daily 7.* They will help you move better. You wake up in the morning and spend 10 minutes right away going through them. These will include:

1. Foot Circle Point and Flexes: 30 seconds point and flex, rotate clockwise: 30 seconds, and counterclockwise: 30 seconds
2. Hip Crossover Stretch: 30 seconds per side,
3. Pelvic Tilts: 30 seconds
4. Birddogs: 30 seconds

5. Arm Glides: 30 seconds
6. Elbow Curls: 30 seconds, and
7. Wall Sit: 30 seconds.

On your Strength Day 1 do Sit to Stands, Reverse Lunges holding a door, Pelvic Tilts, Cats and Dogs, Birddogs, and March in Place.

On Day 3 do Elbow Curls, Stork Stands, Squat Press with dumbbells and a chair, Standard Push-up/or Assisted Push-Up on your knees, Dumbbell Bench Press, Lat Pull Down, and Rowing Machine.

On Day 5, do the entire workout from start to finish.

On Day 2, 4, and 6 you will do cardio days, doing a 30-45 minutes cardio interval routine using the format I described in Chapter 6. Follow the **Daily/Weekly Movement Guide** on the following page for your entire workout schedule.

(If any exercise causes pain, stop doing them and take them out of your workout sequence.) Your goal is to begin to get a kinesthetic sense of how your body feels when you train. You're learning how to move and feel better.

Schedule It Now

Take the next step. How to get started is get your calendar out and schedule your workouts into your mobile calendar like an appointment with your dentist or accountant or doctor. It's as important as any appointment you make for yourself or your family. Why? If you want to be there for your kids, business, extended family, or whatever is truly important to you, you must take care of yourself to be able to give to all the people you listed. Who's going to handle a dying family member better? The man or woman who is continuing to exercise, eat whole foods, and get sleep.

Conversely, the person who uses the situation to burn out, stop exercising, eat fast food, and not sleep? I can guarantee your family wants you to stay healthy and not let your body go to hell in a handbasket.

Daily/Weekly Movement Guide						
*3 days of 30 minute cardiovascular training (**Cvt**) *3 days of strength training (**Stre**) *Daily movement/Body balancing exercises						
Mon	Tue	Wed	Thurs	Fri	Sat	Sun
Stre	**Cvt**	**Stre**	**Cvt**	**Stre**	**Cvt**	**Active Rest**

List three goals for the year and break them down into two-month intervals:

Goal 1:

_____

_____

_____

_____

Goal 2:

_____

_____

_____

_____

Goal 3:

_____

_____

_____

_____

CHAPTER 12

Why I Do What I Do
and You Can, too!

> *"Don't ask yourself what the world needs. Ask yourself what makes you come alive, and go do that, because what the world needs is people who have come alive."*
>
> **— Gil Bailie**

My background and journey defined through health and fitness. Back when I was a young kid, I truly loved to compete, whether it was soccer, basketball, baseball, beach volleyball, hockey, tennis, tackle football on the beach—I just loved to play.

Any sport you could pick, I was interested in doing it. During my high school years my focuses truly became beach volleyball, basketball, indoor volleyball, and soccer.

Freshman year I developed hamstring problems during a growth spurt, where it was difficult to even sprint. I just kind of suffered through it. My sophomore year, I was playing basketball and I felt pretty good.

I started to develop some left shoulder pain later at the end of my sophomore year in volleyball season. Junior year in high school, I started getting tendonitis in my left knee. I started to get tendonitis below my knees my senior year, and by freshman year in college, I had tendonitis all up and down my knees and bone spurs below my knees.

There Is A Way to Get Better

Maybe it seems crazy to think, but I truly believed that there was a way to get myself better. I just felt like with the right training and the right mechanics and the right coaching, someone could help me get there. I didn't think it was surgery, but I looked at that option. I didn't think it was something simple; I just intuitively knew that there was something out there. Before I found Pete Egoscue, I tried everything under the sun. Doctors, orthopedic surgeons, chiropractors, physical therapists, acupressure, acupuncture, and I just couldn't seem to get better. Nothing seemed to work.

When I went to the Egoscue Method, the shift was pretty quick. I was very skeptical, but I was also empowered with the notion of doing corrective movements that were going to change my alignment and change my body to help me feel better. I went through the process, and remarkably, after two and a half years of chronic knee pain, I could run again. I could run on asphalt. I could jump. I could play. I was truly amazed at the quickness and effectiveness of the training.

It motivated me to want to help other people because I felt like, "If this helped me this much, whatever I could find that was going to help me is what I would do to help others for the rest of my life." It turned out to be movement training, and that's what I wanted to learn. That's what I wanted to learn at age 19. I knew it. I knew it back then that this was what I wanted to dedicate myself to. I had overcome massive knee pain, and I wanted to help others who were struggling just like I had struggled.

That's what motivated me to work for Pete at a young age of twenty-one and to get Pete and the Egoscue Method to mentor me. Then that led me to getting my degree at San Diego State, concurrently in kinesiology, where I was already under the process of doing so. Spending nearly five years working at the Egoscue Method, for the formidable years of my life, I can't thank them enough for training me and for the knowledge that I learned there. Being mentored set me on a path of looking for balance and alignment in everything I do.

It set the course of my professional career to think differently. Learning from a marine, who traditionally would say "No pain, no gain," but instead was teaching postural alignment and this idea of listening to your body. He would say, "Pain is an indicator of your body telling you something. Don't fear the pain, but, instead, listen to it."

Those lessons have been so helpful in training myself and my clients through different injuries and helping so many different people through the years. The push for hardcore beat-the-hell-out-of-you training currently popular—it just seems so shortsighted. I enjoy watching the CrossFit games when they come on TV, but it's just not sustainable. I am so grateful for the lessons I learned from Pete those many years ago.

My contribution to the world of health and fitness is successfully combining the notion of correct posture and movement with resistance and strength training. Using strength training as a means to further balance the body.

One of my clients came to me and was tearing up when I told her I was leaving San Diego for my move to Los Angeles to do a tour of duty in inner city school teaching. She stopped me and said, "I want you to know you changed my life."

At twenty-six, I knew what she meant; Pete had changed mine seven years before. I didn't know what to say to that at the time, but I've gotten that response again and again and again through the years, and it makes me feel good to know I can help others. As the Bible says, "Heal the broken hearted, set the captives free."

I have spent the last twenty years of my life dedicating myself to helping others move better. I have so much respect for the individuals who have helped me and encouraged me to learn more. I have been a practitioner of movement training over these many years. I have trained many clients and trainers to think about the alignment of the body and correct movement as a top priority. Healthy joints and functional movement is more than big muscles. I put these ideas into practice every day when we train clients at my personal training fitness studio. They work. As Arnold says, "Reps, reps, reps, you have to put in the work." The key is training smarter, moving better, and building a healthy body, one that is built to last.

Fear vs. Awareness

Smarter training is the answer so many of my clients see and feel after training with us. It's like a veil has been lifted from one's eyes and they can see how their movements or lack of movements affects everything.

Once you are aware of ways to improve your posture and movement, there is a sense of empowerment. You don't have to be in fear of injuring your low back bending down to pick up something off the floor.

The next step is up to you. At the end of the day, it's about learning how to move better and understanding your biomechanics better for a lifetime. There are a lot of good people doing physical therapy, occupational therapy, chiropractic and many others forms of health and medical treatment. The key is you learn for yourself how your body works.

The body has an amazing ability to heal itself if you give it the chance. If you get physical therapy or chiropractic care for a back injury or any specific area of the body, you want to know how to move correctly when you graduate from their care. You're back at the gym, in a class, or outside. What should your squat look like? This is very empowering. Think proper movement for the rest of your life.

When you feel like you can't do something because of pain, excess weight, lack of belief in yourself, I can relate, but I know you *can*. It starts in your mind. I believe in you. Build on what you can do. Someone might say, "I can't run anymore after my knee replacement at sixty. I just can't seem to move like I used to."

What CAN you do? Build on the small things. Hire someone who understands you. Someone who can customize a program to fit your needs. They're out there. I enjoy finding out about my clients, their injuries, challenges, heartbreaks. It all seems to help me find ways to motivate and encourage them to succeed. When you succeed, I succeed.

I pray that you become the person you are designed to be. To become the best version of yourself. You have what it takes. The next step is up to you. Take action and be the healthy person you are designed to be.

To your health,
Your friend,
Bryan Wisdom

ABOUT THE AUTHOR

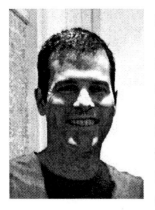 **BRYAN WISDOM** has two decades of experience in the health and fitness industry. He started training college athletes in 1996. He received his B.S. in Kinesiology from San Diego State University and his Master's in Education from Loyola Marymount University. Bryan spent nearly five years training clients in biomechanics at the Egoscue Method exercise therapy company in San Diego, California. He was certified by the NSCA and has worked with NFL, NBA, and professional golfers. He has assisted clients with postural and biomechanical issues and uses exercise and movement to restore the body to proper function. "For me, training is about getting to know my clients, finding the best ways to help them attain their goals."

For the last decade he has served the Mooresville com-munity as owner/operator of Fitness Together Mooresville in North Carolina. During that time he has built a great staff. "All my team members go through a very specific training system, learning posture and corrective movement. It's great to see how much of an impact our trainers make in our client's lives." You may see him out on the lake or a trail doing things that make him come alive. His passions include surfing, wakeboarding, stand-up paddleboarding, trail running, and kiteboarding.

If you would like more information my direct line is (704) 658-1522. Option two: Get a free copy of my Foundation Movements at FTLKN.com.

You can give this book...
To help others
To inspire
To thank
To encourage

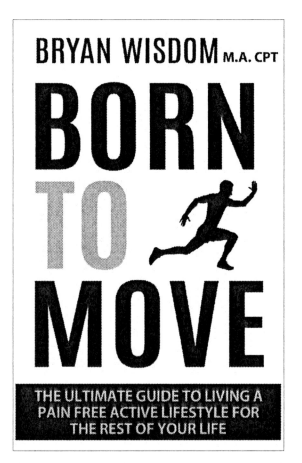

Books are thoughtful gifts that provide a genuine sentiment that other promotional items cannot express. They promote employee discussions and interaction, reinforce an event's meaning or location, and they make a lasting impression. Use this book to say "Thank You" and show people that you care.

Born to Move by Bryan Wisdom is available at **www.amazon.com.**

If you would like more information my direct line is (704) 658-1522. Option two: Get a free copy of my Foundation Movements at FTLKN.com.